# The Compact Workout

Change your life in under 15 minutes a day

A book by Tony Notarianni

*Thank you to all my healers, teachers, friends, and family for guiding me down this path.*

# Foreword

In 2022 I finally gave up exercise as I knew it. I was tired of the countless times I had taken advantage of a stable period in my busy life to embark on a training regimen, to make great progress, and then have it taken away by factors completely out of my control. I did not give up on exercise; I just gave up on my methodology and began from scratch. I stopped thinking "HOW can I find a way to do things the way I KNOW work for me?" Instead, I thought to myself "What can I do NOW? And HOW can I make it SUSTAINABLE?" This resulted in two years of combining study with trial and error, until I finally got into a place that I considered effective enough to share with others.

Of course, there is a major problem with sharing my results which is this: there exists a well substantiated body of research, countless books, and an entire fitness and medical industry devoted to exercise and health. What could I have to offer from an anecdotal perspective?

But let me ask a counter question, if all these things are true, why are so many people not able to take command of their own fitness, at the mercy of factors beyond their control, and often misinformed about the most basic aspects of their own body? I don't know if there is one correct answer to this question, but I can tell you this: the mainstream solution isn't working, and although I cannot guarantee my methodology will work for you, it worked for me, and I suspect with a bit of personalized adaptation it can work for anyone.

And that is the key word here, adaptation. You must adapt yourself, to create a challenging yet sustainable level of daily activity, and a set of dietary changes that will cause your body to adapt, which will result in a difference in how you feel about yourself and change how you interact with the world. The ability to evolve and change with the times is a key element of survival in nature, and so I hope you read this book with this word "adaptation" at the back of your mind. Learn from my lessons and apply them in your life as you see fit.

# Contents

# Introduction

## Who This Book is For

This book is primarily for busy people who want to achieve and maintain a reasonable baseline of fitness without having to dedicate excessive daily time, expense, or thought to it. The ideal reader is someone starting from a baseline of being mostly inactive. This book is not for exercise academics or professionals, athletes, or trainers, or those who intend to achieve results way above a moderate baseline. If you have multiple responsibilities, time constraints, but are willing to put in up to 15 minutes every day to make long term sustainable changes to your body, your mind, and your life in general, then please enjoy this book.

## About the Book

The focus of this book is on how to achieve worthwhile fitness results in a realistic and sustainable schedule. I have condensed the key information from my ongoing fitness journey into a brief journal, followed by a summary, and finally a collection of usable exercises and customizable routines. Rather than delving into detailed explanations, my focus is on laying out the key points simply and clearly so that you can quickly implement your own changes and start seeing results yourself. These results are not just beneficial for the self, but for families, communities, and society.

Reasons for Writing:
1. Sharing My Journey: After speaking to others about my fitness journey, especially those who noticed my changes and wanted to implement their own, I thought it made sense to author a book.

2. Impacting Lives: I genuinely believe that the ideas in this book can change lives for the better. If I can add even a small amount of positive change, it will be worth it.

3. Further Investment: If I generate enough interest, I can invest further and deeper into this topic, having a greater impact on human fitness.

# Understanding Modern Wellness Challenges

In medicine, health conditions are broadly categorized into acute (e.g., a broken arm) and chronic (e.g., arthritis). One major difference is that acute conditions present themselves more easily. If we cast our minds back to the first humans walking the earth, it would be fair to say there were mostly "acute" dangers. Danger could come from environmental exposure, thirst, starvation, accidents, dangerous creatures, and unfortunately, other humans. There were no legal systems, no hospitals, no municipalities, and no infrastructure. Today, it very much depends on where you are, but thankfully, at any point in time, much of the world is peaceful, and technology has lessened these dangers to such a great extent that in many locations we often forget about them entirely.

But what about the more "chronic" dangers plaguing the modern human race? Consider the abundance of foods on the shelves with low fiber and high sugar, ingredients that are overly processed and chemically enhanced, and a food industry that seeks to lower costs by reducing quality and instead maximizing profit through clever marketing.

Or think about the internet and how social media uses highly detailed information about our online activity to target marketing at a subconscious level via algorithms. Consider the addictive nature of online services, curated content, and artificially trended topics. Think about the power of technology to control what we experience, and all the inherent dangers that poses.

Think about all the toxic people who thrive on the ability to reach an entire planet with words designed to deceive, manipulate, and sow negativity. Consider the polarization of ideas, the lack of nuance, and the isolation of interactions caused by grouping people by politics, religion, lifestyle, and other factors. Think about the pollution in the air, water, and soil. Think about the impacts of invasive species, the rapid spread of diseases, and human-caused disasters.

Think about the disinformation that encapsulates all of this, so that we do not know exactly who to listen to or what to believe. There are a million pieces of advice for dealing with modern living, especially online. "One weird trick," "the secret nobody wants you to know," "the top X strategies for success," and other cliché marketing gimmicks.

When it comes back to fitness, everywhere you look, there are health/exercise products, supplements, superfoods, obscure exercise regimes, and transformation programs to sign up for. Unfortunately, although a number of these have their place, there is no silver bullet that works for everyone. However, it can be an exploitative, money-making business model that, rather than helping us, feeds back into the list of chronic concerns facing the modern human.

We humans may have advanced our ability to deal with the acute, but we have done so by increasing our exposure to the chronic. In such a toxic environment, it is a miracle that most of us still function as human beings and operate in societies that support each other. The expectation that we could all somehow take great care of ourselves can sometimes be overwhelming, riddled with distraction, plagued by disinformation, and doomed by false expectations. That is, unless you can make the most of the most critical and limited resources of all: time and money. This will be the key strategy in this book.

# The Power of Motivation: Finding Your Why

Before moving forward, I want to discuss the importance of motivation. Without the correct motivation, anything is doomed to fail. Think about a person who wants to get healthy so that they look more attractive, hoping to find a romantic partner. This is indeed strong motivation because sex is a biologically built-in driver for most humans. The person may engage very strongly by exercising and dieting to achieve the killer physique they want.

It works, and the combination of their personality and appearance enables them to find that partner they were looking for. Now what? If the motivation were to get that partner, once they have that partner, the motivation would diminish. Or even worse, they might become insecure, and this might jeopardize the recently established relationship.

If the motivation is short-term, then your progress will be as well. It is best to find motivation that is lifelong, compelling, and well thought out.

Examples of Lasting Motivation:
- A desire to continue enjoying physical activities well into old age.
- Increasing your chances of being around to support loved ones.
- Being able to function more fully in daily life.
- Overcoming or stabilizing a chronic ailment.
- Wanting to be more productive in society and requiring less support.

# The Compact Workout

The important thing is to understand why what you are doing is important to you and constantly remind yourself of this source of motivation.

# Case Study: My Exercise Life Rollercoaster

As a young child, I was never particularly adept at organized sports. In fairness to myself, it was not something with which I was surrounded. Despite, by the age of seven, having lived in four countries and attending multiple schools, there had not been much emphasis on the subject. Once I found myself in places where sport (particularly soccer) was considered important, I was never able to catch up. My family also were not participants or spectators of sport, so I was at the mercy of the public education system, which failed to bridge the gap over the next eleven years.

Physically, though, I was active. By the age of nine, I would spend hours in the local park making every conceivable use of the local playground, climbing trees, playing hiding games, and leaping from high places. I enjoyed pushing myself, wondering how many laps of the monkey bars I could achieve without stopping, and how high I could come off the swing and land on my feet. When I was twelve, a friend of mine asked if I wanted to start karate classes with him. Although most karate classes at that age were circuit training and stretching, my body felt amazing, and I continued attending for the next two years. At the age of fifteen I found other martial arts to enjoy which I continue to practice to this day.

I also asked my parents for dumbbells, and later a barbell and weights bench for my birthday gifts during my mid-teens. I found that after coming home from school, the stress relief of exercise was incredibly beneficial. When I was seventeen, I found employment at a public sports facility and became a pool lifeguard. I also had free access to the gym, and before long, I was swimming laps and getting stronger by lifting heavier weights. Somehow, I had found my own outlet for exercise, and although I did not have a sports team or a competition to enter,

The Compact Workout

I just knew that it was something I enjoyed and needed to do to feel complete.

I ended up studying sport as part of my higher education, the other class members were confused about this as they were all active in sport, whereas I was just active. At the age of eighteen, a typical week consisted of four hours of weight training, one hour of swimming, five hours of martial arts of varying intensity, and up to ten hours of walking everywhere. Almost twenty hours of activity, with full-time studying, part-time working, and partying on the weekends.

| Age | High intensity | Medium | Low | Health (approx.) |
|---|---|---|---|---|
| 18 | 5hrs | 5hrs | 10hrs | Weight 156 lb.<br>BP 120/70<br>HR 60 |

When I left for university to pursue a degree in sports science, everything changed around me. I no longer had as much money to spend on food, I had to do more for myself, I had no free access to a gym or a pool, and the number of hours required to study increased significantly. I had less places to go, less energy to walk, and the local environment was hostile anyway. In the space of under two years, I got sick several times: chickenpox, influenza, German measles, and on my twentieth birthday, my knee was so swollen with an infection I could not bend my leg.

I did enjoy a period at the university fencing club, I still occasionally had flurries of exercise, but the mindset always seemed to be one of frustration and telling myself I would figure this out when the situation got better. And of course, the situation was never better.

By the time I graduated, I had lost all the strength I had gained previously. I felt tired most of the time with truly little stamina, and in martial arts too, I found myself more susceptible to injury and less competitive. It was the flu that had taken the most out of me, and I found myself spending more time using this recent technology called the internet and less time taking care of myself.

| Age | High intensity | Medium | Low | Health (approx.) |
|---|---|---|---|---|
| 22 | 0hrs | 3hrs | 5hrs | Weight 150lb<br>BP 125/75<br>HR 65 |

After graduation, I entered the workforce and started to earn an income. I had money now, but I just felt so unfit. I started running in the evening, and for a while, I ran for miles every night, in the rain, in the dark, even in the snow. But then I decided to go to night school as I really wanted to get a career in technology. I was also in a series of relationships, and my girlfriends wanted to spend time with me, but not working out with me, and I found it a point of contention most of the time. In one job I strained my back moving office furniture, I could not believe it, what was happening to me?

Eventually, I got my new technology job and what would be a multi-decade career had started, but I had to commute by car which took more time out of the day. I sometimes ran with friends during my lunch hour, but often my days were spent sitting in a car, or at a desk, finally reaching home only to have other tasks in front of me.

It was very frustrating; every time I thought I would finally get to the point where I could get back to the energetic, healthy lifestyle I had enjoyed, something changed. I joined gyms and quit, shuffled schedules, tried eating differently, but no matter what I did, it just felt like I was getting further and further away from where I wanted to be, which is where I used to be. So, I spent more time online, more time playing video games, more time watching TV and movies. These are things that have increasingly become more convenient and immersive over time, and not impacted by the same restricting factors as an exercise regimen. Of course, this helped neither me, my career, nor my relationships.

| Age | High intensity | Medium | Low | Health (approx.) |
| --- | --- | --- | --- | --- |
| 25 | 1hr | 2hrs | 2hrs | Weight 165lb<br>BP 125/75<br>HR 70 |

By the time I was in my mid-thirties I had a recurring bad back, degrading knee strength, a growing waistline, and decreased circulation. My career had led me to a place where I was working long hours, often on call and working through the night. I had lived and worked in Asia and was now living in a new country (the USA), however, I found that my immigration status left me much at the mercy of my employers and their clients.

I was still doing martial arts and the occasional gym, but I was beginning to wonder how long I would be able to maintain any level of fitness or activity. To make matters worse I fell badly at one point and injured my clavicle. I was referred to a chiropractor who assessed me and discovered I had a serious misalignment of my hips, tightness in my ribs, and neck issues.

Moving to the US added a lot of carbohydrates to my diet, which caused me to put an unhealthy amount of weight on. I was starting to feel more hungry, more tired, less able to concentrate, and this began to make me feel increasingly powerless and depressed.

| Age | High intensity | Medium | Low | Health (approx.) |
| --- | --- | --- | --- | --- |

| 35 | 0hrs | 3hrs | 2hrs | Weight 185lb<br>BP 130/80<br>HR 70 |
|---|---|---|---|---|

Luckily around this time I began regular yoga in the evening and at weekends, and after my first class it gave me this positive healthy feeling that I had not felt for a long time. It was incredibly beneficial, and it gave me a new lease on life. Between ongoing chiropractic treatment and regular yoga, I suddenly found myself in a much better place than I had been in for several years. I was waking up two hours earlier and using a local gym. I was at the gym five hours a week, doing martial arts three hours a week, and about two hours a week of yoga. Ten hours of exercise a week, it had taken me twenty years to get back to half the level of exercise I was doing originally. There was just one problem, it did not leave much time for everything else, and I had a lot going on.

I still remember the call from my dermatologist. I had noticed a strange spot on my leg, it looked like an insect bite, or a squeezed zit, but it was not healing. My doctor recommended I get it looked at and at first the dermatologist seemed confident it was nothing, he took a biopsy and sent it off. "I will call you in a week if there are any issues, if you don't hear from me by then it's nothing." A week later I was wrapping up my workday and the phone rang; it was not good news for two reasons. Firstly, it was cancer, secondly it was not a typical case, and his office did not have the ability to deal with it. I was referred from there to a surgeon.

After the call I went to tell my fiancé, we were planning our wedding, getting excited about starting a family and building a life together. Now this. We tried not to think about it too much while we waited for my consultation. Fortunately, after speaking with an expert, I had lucked out, the cancer, although a nasty one, had been caught early and was very accessible.

The Compact Workout

Before long I was in surgery and had some skin and a part of my leg removed. After this I was mobile quickly, but although I was moving around it was some time before I could put pressure on my leg or stretch in certain directions. I was so relieved that my wedding and indeed my life was soon back on track. It was though another reminder of how fragile my fitness regimen was, it took a long time to get back into the flow of things and it was not long before I reached my next crossroads.

Leading up to the wedding I was exercising again, I would hit the gym early before the equipment got crowded. I would run a mile on the treadmill as fast as I could as a warmup, reaching my record of 6:02 minutes. I then did a gross motor movement (deadlift or rows), (bench or shoulder press), (squat or leg press), followed by some core/bodyweight exercises, then a prolonged cool down and stretch. Often this would take over an hour. I started making gains again and was lifting over half of what I had been as a teenager. I felt rather good, and I was pleased with my progress. Yoga complimented my routine, and I was mentally feeling better.

| Age | High intensity | Medium | Low | Health (approx.) |
|-----|----------------|--------|------|------------------|
| 40 | 3hrs | 3hrs | 3hrs | Weight 175lb<br>BP 125/75<br>HR 65 |

I still remember the last time I did such a workout; it was the morning before my first child was born. And what an incredible and life-changing experience that was. I quickly learned though that in terms of my ability to sustain a training regimen, things had changed. Now there was a tiny helpless baby on a feeding cycle of just a few hours. So even if I forced myself to work out, I really did not have the same energy or the ability to recover afterwards. My brain also changed. I had avoided babies my whole life and had no knowledge of how to care for one, and suddenly I was learning at a rapid rate, and realizing the depth of responsibilities that come with it. My aggression levels, my ability to focus, and my attitudes to life were all shifting about making it difficult to focus the way I used to.

My priorities had to change, time was limited dramatically, and availability to exercise became highly inconsistent. Training the body the way I was used to in order to make gains requires consistency, capacity for planning, time to execute, and adequate recovery. It seemed like I had none of these. The irony was that having children certainly made me want to fight to be a better provider overall, and that included being in decent shape, but I could not see a way to sustain my personal fitness yet. I changed jobs, I changed houses, and during this time also found out we were having another baby!

I was active, packing and moving boxes, fixing up a house to sell, running after a toddler, doing odd jobs and errands. It kept my heart pumping but my body increasingly ached. My back hurt, my neck hurt, my knees hurt, and I felt increasingly less able to physically take care of my family which was affecting my mental state as a husband and father.

My only exercise came via my visits to a chiropractor who also shared an office with a physical therapist. I had been given some unwelcome news, x-rays showed I had developed some cervical and lumbar kyphosis. This was determined to be manageable but would require constant work and would never reverse. Before or after chiropractic adjustment I was given exercises to warm up, stretch, mobilize, and strengthen stabilizing muscles. It felt so good to be doing something, and even if just for a couple of times a month I could get anywhere from 30-60 mins of rehabilitating exercise. I also had someone coach me and ensured good form throughout.

The key benefit was that I learned specific exercises for targeting the weaker supportive muscles that tend to atrophy when we neglect them, and compensate them, resulting in unnecessary joint pain and in some cases injury. The negative aspect of all this was that I could not afford to maintain the appointments and had limited options to do anything in between. Instead, I studied the exercises in terms of how they felt and how my body responded.

My second child was born during the pandemic, it was such a surreal time for our family. A year afterwards we were dealing with some mysterious health issues, none of the doctors knew what to do, and neither did I. Financially we were struggling, mentally and physically we were exhausted, and to make matters worse the children were also going through issues of their own. We did not have a lot of access to support, and we were paying a lot of money for babysitting and preschool.

It was also a very tense time at work and in addition to my personal life I also had to juggle a multitude of other tasks. It was completely unmanageable. As for the children, I took them out every chance I could. The backyard, the beach, the park, a walk, anything. It was great for them and the best I could do for exercise and mental health.

This went on for some time, and just as we started to get out of it, we found out baby three was on the way. At this point I knew, any ideas about gym, running, yoga, or any of my personal health and fitness goals were going to be on the backburner for years. I might be in my sixties before I could even think about it again.

| Age | High intensity | Medium | Low | Health (approx.) |
|---|---|---|---|---|
| 18 | 5hrs | 5hrs | 10hrs | Weight 156 lb.<br>BP 120/70<br>HR 60 |
| 22 | 0hrs | 3hrs | 5hrs | Weight 150lb |

| | | | | BP 125/75<br>HR 65 |
|---|---|---|---|---|
| 25 | 1hr | 2hrs | 2hrs | Weight 165lb<br>BP 125/75<br>HR 70 |
| 35 | 0hrs | 3hrs | 2hrs | Weight 185lb<br>BP 130/80<br>HR 70 |
| 40 | 3hrs | 3hrs | 3hrs | Weight 175lb<br>BP 135/80<br>HR 60 |
| 45 | 0hrs | 3hrs | 2hrs | Weight 175lb<br>BP 140/85<br>HR 65 |

# Why My Story Is Useful

As you can see, despite all my desire to do exercise, which I enjoyed, and five years of higher education studying sport, I was constantly putting it on the backburner of life. Whether it was my career, relationships, health, or personal responsibilities, I could never sustain a regular pattern of exercise beyond a few months at a time. The result was very demoralizing, despite all my intentions, and invested time, I had nothing to show for it. My body was still weak and aging, my health was deteriorating, and I was struggling to keep up despite having more responsibilities than ever before.

It has been convenient in my early life to think of people who do not exercise as lazy, but I think more likely they have just given up on it. It conflicts with life, it is not sustainable, it costs money, and it is just too hard. If I failed to be consistent, with all my knowledge and intention, how could everyone else be expected to motivate themselves constantly? I could see how easy it is to develop habits that are not healthy, and how those activities are getting more powerfully alluring than ever. In a sense, that was the first lesson. Humility. Exercising one day, or for a few weeks, is easy. But keeping your entire life active in a sustainable and meaningful way? That is hard and ironically getting harder than ever as I was beginning to realize myself.

I had reached a crossroads, in one direction I could keep trying and failing to take control of my fitness the same way I had for decades, in another direction I could just accept the hand I was dealt and give up, I didn't like either of these options anymore. Suddenly it occurred to me, "what if I needed to redefine what exercise and fitness meant to me now. The me I am now, in this time." And "what if instead of thinking of time as a barrier, I turn it on itself and use it somehow." But how?

# My Discovery Log

Where to start?

One day in 2022 while I was working from home I had a short break between calls. And I thought "what if I could figure out a way to train in a short amount of time?" The problem I faced was I knew that I needed a warmup, but also the intensity needed to be enough to make me feel worked out. By the time I warmed up, it was time to go back to work. But without a warmup, it will not feel good, and I might hurt myself. Also, what exercise to do? My whole body needs a balanced workout, so what exercises should I do?

I thought about my body type. I am lean and thin, built for endurance, but also have a good history of explosive tensile strength exercises. But when it came to 10-20 repetitions my muscles always burned out quickly. I reasoned that I liked heavy weights and endurance due to avoidance. I was doing the things I enjoyed and felt comfortable with, rather than the things that felt challenging. I decided to focus on my weakness, intermediate endurance.

At first, I considered just doing three main exercises. Push-ups, squats, and crunches. I thought, well if I cannot do heavy, I will just do more repetitions. I set a ridiculous vague goal of reaching a high number of reps: 100 push-ups, 200 squats, and 150 crunches. I did as many as I could in a set of each and then the next day, I did the same. At first it was fun, in fact for a few days I improved each day, but after that I began to waver around the same numbers each day, sometimes getting worse. So, I started breaking them into sets and taking more rest in between.

Within just two weeks I hit a wall. The wall was not actually the ability to make progress to my goal, it was the investment required to keep making those gains. I now needed to do other exercises and stretches to balance out the exercises I had chosen, I needed more warming up, and, most of all, I needed something I did not have. Time. I was seeing the pattern again.

## Tabata with Squat Burpees

I formulated a plan. If time was my limitation, then I would take control of it and limit my own time. I would do timed exercises. But what timing regimen should I use? I investigated different timing methods, and one leapt out at me. Tabata was originally designed for cyclists and used the idea of intense intervals and rest periods of specific durations. Three sets of intervals to be precise.

I did not have a bike, or any equipment, but I figured I would pick a full body exercise. I chose the jumping squat burpee and one day after work I set the stopwatch and did it. Well honestly, I did one set and gassed out. And I was so sore the following days. I kept doing this every other day and eventually did a full round, and even a second round. I was super focused on progressing, but instead of feeling great I felt terrible.

The issue was I lacked any warmup, mobility work, and there was nothing to encourage good form. I was just leaping about and straining my joints. It was brutal. Back to the drawing board.

## Tuning the Times and Increasing the Variety

I decided that true tabata was just too long, too restrictive, and too harsh, and I needed to mix things up. I analyzed the timings and decided I wanted the whole thing to last under 15 minutes. I came to this number because I analyzed my day, and I found that realistically among all my responsibilities 15 minutes was a sweet spot of opportunity.

I also observed that sometimes I was so stressed and compressed that I might spend 10-20 minutes just listening to music, scrolling on social media, or soaking in the shower. Although just standing there, letting warm water ease my muscles, and letting the water drown out my senses was therapeutic it seemed a wasted opportunity. I decided to shorten and earn my showers.

I also used a trick of association. When I went to take a shower, I made myself think "earn it." And this way I developed the habit of exercising every time I took a shower. I would spend 10-15 mins exercising and 2-5 mins quickly showering.

I had now established a daily pattern of exercise. I tried regular basic exercises like push-ups, sit-ups, and squats. This did seem to help at first, but I did feel myself getting tight again.

## Stretching the Spine and the Hips

About 15 years prior I was introduced to the Japanese system of Makko Ho. At a basic level it is a series of four primary postures you must relax in while maintaining good form, symmetry, and attitude. These four positions at a surface level appear as the butterfly stretch, the forward fold, the forward fold with split, and the yoga hero pose.

The founder of the Makko Ho system used these positions to restore his body after a stroke, having been told he would be bedridden the remainder of his life. And there is a great deal more to this system than meets the eye. The main aspect that I find challenging is the discipline to do a little bit every day.

As I wanted my 15 mins of exercise a day to pump blood and develop better and stronger movement, I was not keen to sacrifice that time for "stretching". Yet, I also felt sore after exercise and wanted to gain good flexibility. I also felt the importance of hip and spine health that Makko Ho promotes, especially with my back diagnosis.

As I thought about this conflict, I realized the key difference between the two was that when "exercising" I needed to focus and not distracted. Doing circuits, I had to be conscious of time, form, and the sequence of exercises. Makko Ho, on the other hand, I could practice while listening to a podcast or watching TV. And so, I started to do it in the evening when the children were asleep, usually spending time with my wife watching TV, or taking 10-15 mins with my headphones listening to educational material or just relaxing music.

Note: I have spent many wonderful years studying yoga, and fully recommend this kind of practice to anyone. In fact, when I had more time on my hands, I would attend two or three classes a week and became proficient in some challenging forms. However, this was not an option in recent years.

# Pushups Challenge

In 2023 I was contacted online by St Jude's hospital, they were targeting specific demographics I assume and asking people to take part in a challenge. 2800 pushups in February, or one hundred push-ups per day. By now you must know that I love to try and solve multiple problems at once. One was motivation, the next was focus, and finally commitment.

By doing something for a kid's charity, once I signed up, I felt constantly motivated by their needs. As the goal was noticeably clear, I simply focused on meeting my goal and counting my daily totals. As people started to sponsor me, I could NOT back out. I was going to do this.

It was also an excellent chance to observe myself and others joining the challenge as a psychological experiment. It became rapidly apparent that many had no idea what they signed up for, others were only there to promote themselves or their business. I decided not to film myself performing pushups, I expected my sponsors to trust me with counting. Filming felt like it would take too much effort and time anyway.

I learned quickly that I could easily do one hundred pushups in a day, as a young man I achieved over seventy in one set, so I was not overly surprised. But after a few days I noticed two things, my body did not like doing the same thing every day without a break, yet my mind got increasingly fanciful ideas about where I would be in a month. In fact, I ended up peaking at around forty reps per set in the middle of the month, but by the end of the challenge I was operating in the range of 20-30 pushups for my main sets. I was convinced I would be cranking out 100 a set by then.

I also learned, thanks to advice from other challengers, that it was best to double up on one day, and then take a rest day. This allowed my body to rest but required even more reps on my workdays. I was surprised how much my body rebelled, and how soreness would not go away even after two days.

At the time I had two toddlers and a baby running around so it was hard to do two hundred pushups in one session with adequate rests between sets. Sometimes my kids even climbed on my back, which was funny but reduced my reps. I had to spread my sets throughout the day. Ten here, twenty there, two sets of thirty later, and so on.

The expectation, the reality. The need to spread the work, the need for rest days in between. The progress towards the goal vs the progress of performance. These distinctions became clearer towards the end, and after completing the challenge I felt ready for a change in myself and my strategy.

## Spreading the Routines

After the pushup challenge, I was beyond convinced that I needed three components for my routine:

1) exercises to mobilize my hips and spine - so I could do more with my body for longer, and as a quick warmup.
2) strengthen my core and upper body - I knew that my core was too weak and causing back issues as well as impacting every other exercise I did, I also knew that my upper body strength had to increase.
3) condition my legs and hips - I wanted to hit some of the stabilizer muscles, and as a martial artist to have better kicks.

I divided my Tabata routine into three cycles to match this. It gave me about 4 mins to work on each area including rest intervals. At first, I needed more rest interval time, not to rest but simply to remember and set up for the next exercise. Eventually I came down to 23 seconds of work, 7 seconds rest/setup, and an extra 20 seconds between cycles.

This gave me eight exercises per cycle, which I thought would provide enough variability but potentially meant changing the routine every day and tracking what I had done previously. Mobility exercises alone involved more movements than I had time for and that was a problem.

Luckily about this time I came across an interesting concept, some PTs were teaching combined mobility exercises. That is instead of just working one movement you would hit two or three areas at once in the same exercise. I determined that I could usually manage 8-10 steady movements in a twenty-three second set hitting multiple movement patterns at the same time. As a result, I was able to begin every session with the same warmup set, and then I just had to choose my upper body/core and leg exercises. Which evolved as I will later explain.

# X Ray Results

As I was embarking on my exercises and stretching most nights, I certainly began to feel a bit better. I was doing something every day, I had a stronger core, I was more flexible, and I felt less pain in the mornings, or after exertions. I was curious though if all my work was having any impact on my posture and spine related conditions.

I spoke to my chiropractor, and he said that we could redo my x-rays, but both he and the other doctor explained that these things are usually irreversible. A week or two later I got the results, and much to everyone's surprise slight curvature had returned to my neck and lumbar area. It was another sign that things were heading in a good direction.

# Commuting Hacks

During this entire process I was headhunted by a recruiter for an open position at a large corporation. The new role required regular commuting to New York city which at first seemed quite daunting. Almost a 2-hour trip each way, into my already busy schedule. Those days seemed like a write off, I could not even get 15 minutes to do my routine, and I sometimes had little energy to stretch at night although my body regretted it if I skipped it.

At the time there seemed to be a growing number of safety concerns in the city, and I was also conscious of the time spent waiting on platforms rather than riding a connecting train. So, I decided to speed walk everywhere. It became something of a game, dodging the crowds, timing the trains, I shaved up to 20 minutes from my morning commute by just walking faster. Getting extra steps and increasing my heart rate gave me a new source of exercise–the best kind.

One day the office lobby was packed with people waiting for elevators and I had to get upstairs quickly for a meeting. I noticed someone entering the door to the stairwell and followed. As I passed the door a small sign read that the stairs were available in the morning and at lunchtime. I walked up to my floor and suddenly felt my lack of fitness. I decided to use the stairs every single day after that. Pretty soon I was bounding up the stairs each morning and still cooling down from exertion by the time I reached my desk or meeting.

As a result of these modifications, I found that on commuting days I got a different kind of exercise, but it was still exercise.

## Resistance Bands

My exercises involved body weight exercises at first, but I had a couple of exercise bands lying around which I tried to incorporate in my routine. It seemed simple enough, by using the bands I was able to do arm curls, upright rows, shoulder press, and add resistance to my squats. The bands varied in resistance and after a few weeks I found that although the resistance was no longer that great, I enjoyed the blood flow and felt benefits in the surrounding connective tissues of the joints.

After some time, I remember taking my oldest daughter to a birthday party. At one point, while I was carrying her, she gave me a cup of juice just at the moment I needed to put her down. Without thinking I began lowering my 40lb daughter gently down onto the bench with one arm while holding a cup in my other hand. As I was doing it, I started to wonder what I was doing. I was convinced I would hurt my back, or strain my arm, or pull something in my shoulder and spill the drink everywhere. Nothing happened. I did not think too much about it at the time, but I was surprised enough to remember it.

It was a little later that I understood the science of resistance bands. Bands apply the most resistance at the extent of the stretch, and the least resistance towards their rest position. That means that when you perform an exercise such as an arm curl, if the other end of the band is under your feet, then the maximum resistance will be when your hand is up at your shoulder. This is variable resistance exercise, as opposed to static resistance exercise. Now in terms of cramming maximum effort into a small workout that suddenly became an appealing principle. It also clearly engaged the muscles in a way that helped protect them.

Using this principle, I made sure that my entire movement was encountering suitable resistance, with the harder part of the exercise encountering less resistance, and the easier part encountering more resistance. This applied both on the way up and the way down. Usually it might feel that three to five sets of an exercise are needed to really push yourself, but with strong bands I found that one or two sets was quite enough to feel a bit of manageable resistance, with less time taken, less chance of injury, and less soreness in the following days.

These bands were good for doing light resistance on days when I did not really want to push myself too hard. More on that later.

## Pull Ups and Body Weight

The Compact Workout

Everything was starting to go well, and after a few months I was doing a nice variety of exercises daily, cramming a number of exercises into a small window of time, and obtaining a range of benefits that improved my mental outlook and physical sense of wellbeing.

I now shifted focus from movement and stabilization to making actual gains. I considered the following to be gains, increasing the number of repetitions, increasing the resistance of the exercise, or moving to a more challenging version of the exercise. It was at this time that I also started to think about which muscle groups were not getting enough work.

My body weight was enough for a good range of upper body exercises hitting my core, chest, back of my arms, and parts of my shoulders. For my legs I was able to hit the smaller stabilizing groups, and even the major muscles like the glutes got some exercise. The main issue was my back and my biceps, the bands I had just did not give enough resistance. The solution I produced for this was to purchase a pull-up bar.

At first, I could not even do one good pull-up, having not tried for several years, I could only manage a couple of chin-ups. After several weeks, this number grew, and I was soon doing alternate sets of three for my eight-set circuit. I experimented by super setting with other exercises, or front loading the pull-ups. I found I could do six to start with but tired out quickly. I was on a plateau.

I wanted to be able to do more in a set. At least ten I thought. As I was thinking about this, I looked in the mirror and asked myself why this was so important to me. How did it fit in with my goals, was it worth pushing and injuring myself? I thought about how I felt compared to months and months prior, how much better things were. But then I looked again. I still had a belly, not a huge one, but on my slender frame it was noticeable.

It was so obvious, if I wanted to increase my pull-ups I had to decrease my excess body fat. But how? I had never really studied diets and nutrition in detail, nor did I understand biology that well. It was time to address this.

## Exercise and Weight

When I was at university studying sport science I had paid attention to the mechanical aspects of movement, and physiology, but my knowledge of nutrition was limited. From my perspective at that age, diet was not an issue, I was slim, I was active, and I was young. I often ate unhealthy meals with no observable consequence. As a result, I did not study any further.

Then there I was, trying to get off this elongated rollercoaster pattern of exercise, and wondering if exercise was the be all and end all of my health and day to day performance. I was not sure anymore what expectations were realistic. So, I decided to study, listening to podcasts and videos as I washed dishes, reading articles on my phone while riding public transport, or listening to interviews while driving.

As I dug into content on the subject something kept coming up. Exercise does not make you lose weight. This went against a lot of what I had come to believe growing up, and even after a university degree in sport science. Surely burning calories and increasing muscle mass would result in you dropping fat? It seemed preposterous to think otherwise.

The counter argument was people who exercise simply get hungrier and eat more. And if they do not it can be quite unhealthy. As I thought about it, I remembered how little energy is burned by the body in a 10K vs how much is in a single candy bar. I never really delved into this before but as I thought about what had been happening to me over the previous months it rang true.

I was exercising for 15 mins daily, had increased some muscle mass, and had a slightly increased metabolism during and post workouts. Did I really expect that to magically burn significant fat? And it was also true, I sometimes ate more because of working out.

So now I knew that I had to deal with dieting, because even if I were in better mechanical shape the extra weight would hinder performance and counter the health benefits and longevity for which I was aiming. Little did I know that it was just the tip of an iceberg that could be a book all on its own.

## The Gut

The first area of interest I found was gut health. A lot of scientists and doctors were talking about the importance of a healthy gut, and I started to see the gut as something I needed to support. Online there were all manner of products and ideas around gut health, foods to eat, foods not to eat.

Often this advice conflicted, but the best piece of advice I received was to ensure variety, especially natural plant-based sources of food. A second key component was to include naturally fermented and probiotic foods as part of daily life. Thirdly by increasing fiber intake I was able to make life easier for my gut. Seeing the gut as a similar concept to a muscle, which can be constantly worked, was another key insight.

When I started to do this, I certainly felt improvement in gut function, and that was a start. It may have reduced bloating and even improved my mental outlook. But I knew I had more to learn. I had also started to develop rosacea and all my research into that also pointed to diet.

# Sugar

Of course, sugar has always been something I knew was bad for me, it rots your teeth, it makes you feel overly energized, and then makes you crash. I was not eating a lot of candies, and I usually went for plain dark chocolate with little sugar added. I did not think I was eating that much sugar.

I knew about glycemic indexes though and knew that certain foods release sugars into your system faster than others. It all came down to something called calorie availability, and this meant not only did each food have different amounts of sugar in them, but they also had distinct types of sugars, and depending on any preparation could result in different amounts of sugar released into the system at different rates.

Now here comes the new part, when there is a certain level of sugar in your system, insulin kicks in to stop your body having a hyperglycemic event. In basic terms substantial amounts of sugar can cause cells to shut down until insulin does its job. What happened next was the missing part for me, insulin takes this sugar and stores it in your body. Some sugar being stored in muscles or other organs, and the rest to fat cells.

My growing belly fat was not specifically the result of eating too much food or exercising too little. It was a gradual result of my body consuming calories that released too quickly for my body to process them, and the fat was my body saving my life through an insulin response. It should also be noted that the spikes in blood sugar also cause long term accumulative cell damage which results in premature aging and overall stress on the immune system. And each spike is followed by a crash, resulting in fatigue, cravings, and irritability.

Once I understood this it completely revolutionized my perspective on diet. I saw the ridiculous faddishness of so many diets and realized that spikes must be avoided as much as reasonably possible.

# Reducing Spikes

I had often heard debates about breakfast over the years, with everything from it being the most important meal of the day, to skipping it entirely. The meaning of breakfast of course being to break the nightly fast when we are sleeping rather than eating. This means we can break the cycle of glucose spikes from the day before and begin a fresh new day. Part of waking up appears to be a hormonal release of organ stored energy into the bloodstream, like a battery starter for the body.

What I was doing however was I am sure what others in the western world tend to do, I was supplementing my glucose release with ingested glucose. Orange juice, large bowls of cereal, and if I was hungry, toast. I would then be sitting at a desk for a day and feeling hungry by mid-morning. I would have caffeine and something sweet before a large filling calorie laden lunch. I would then spend the afternoon trying to stay awake, and finally eat dinner that consisted mostly of meat and starch with few to no vegetables.

I was spiking and crashing my blood sugar levels all day long and doing nothing with that excess energy. Day by day my waistband was growing, I had to buy new pants, I could not wear fitted clothes, and when I tried to exercise with body weight, I felt sluggish and tired easily. It all started to become clearer.

In my case I completely stopped fruit juices and instead only ate whole raw fruit throughout the day. For breakfast I ate plain whole yogurt/kefir with berries, and an egg. If I had bread, it was the minimum and after I ate yogurt. This meant that I was not skipping breakfast, but the glucose I was ingesting was minimal and encased in fiber. I was not extending my nightly fast, just the glucose aspect of it. Now I would go from 9pm to at least 10:30am without significant spikes, over 12 hours a day where I was not stressing my body.

Mid-morning I would often have coffee and a snack, I gradually moved the coffee to right after breakfast, and the snack if I needed one became fruit, nuts, or even seeds. Sometimes I ate chocolate, but it felt like a choice rather than a habit. I drank water, or sometimes apple cider infused drinks throughout the day.

At lunch I would eat two kinds of meals. One choice was a salad, my favorite being Greek style with tomatoes, olives, and feta cheese. Oil and vinegar dressing along with salt and pepper was all I needed. I would sometimes add extra protein, but this was a good go-to choice for me. I just had to make sure to keep fresh tomatoes handy and the prep time was minutes.

Another lunch meal was leftovers with a twist. For example, I may have made chicken, vegetables, and rice for a meal the night before. But rather than eat this as a meal I would supplement it with kimchi or sauerkraut. I might add nuts or seeds, in either case I would reduce the rice to compensate. As a result, I gave my gut fermented food, lowered my glucose spikes, and added some extra flavor to my meal.

Dinner was the main family meal of the day, so rather than try and change what we eat, I just changed how I ate it. I made extra vegetables compared to before and increased my ratio of those while decreasing the carbs. I used food ordering when I ate, prioritizing vegetables, protein, and then carbohydrates to further reduce spikes. I also tried to be active immediately after a meal, doing dishes, playing with my kids, taking out the trash, anything on my feet.

In the evening, I tried to avoid snacking, but if I was hungry, I would focus on raw foods and avoid anything processed. I was not religious about this, just like with my exercise regimen I wanted to be realistic and think about my motivations and goals. I considered myself to be trending towards a better direction health wise, rather than letting myself trend towards a worse place. It was the net result that mattered not the individual days.

After doing this diet modification for a couple of months it became second nature, I felt more energetic, less bloated, more focused, and simply better. I went for an annual checkup and was surprised to see that my blood pressure, which had been creeping up over the last few decades, had dropped to where it was in my early twenties. My oncologist was also surprised by my change after not having seen me for six months. I had not really noticed any change but when I checked my belt, I was now tightening it many inches further than before.

Finally, I got on the scales and realized I had lost about 12lbs. I decided to go for it with my pull-ups and see. I did eleven in a set. It was my best in almost 30 years. My rosacea improved, and I was able to wear clothes I had thought of discarding. Above all, I knew that I had potentially extended the life and use of my body.

# Kettlebell

Now that I had developed my routine over several months, I was feeling quite good. I had modified my habits, my diet, and my approach using researched and realistically implemented methods. As a result, I was physically and mentally healthier, in better shape, and able to perform better in a multitude of ways.

## The Compact Workout

I began to wonder though; can I take this further? Do not get me wrong, I was pleased with what I had achieved, it was certainly an accomplishment but there were a few things I wanted to add to my routines. One of these components was more resistance exercises.

Up to this point I had used bodyweight and bands, which worked very well, but I felt that free weight exercises would complement my workouts. I did not really want to invest in a lot of complicated equipment and so I thought about exploring kettlebells. I had only used them for physical therapy exercises in the past and intended to do more. I was thinking of them primarily as working the supporting muscles rather than the major muscle groups.

I was not ready to invest so I put it on the Christmas wish list, and on Christmas day I received a solid 45 lb. kettlebell. 45lb felt heavier than I remembered, I had often changed this exact weight as a disc on an Olympic barbell over the years, it never felt that heavy. Now suddenly it felt like a strain, and I wondered how this was going to work out. I would advise a lighter weight if you were going to follow my lead in this program. 25lb would have been more appropriate.

I started with full body exercises; squats and lunges, followed by some swings. I soon realized this was a weight that was going to hit my major muscle groups so I started to think how including reps in a circuit could add to my routine without injuring me. I decided that my pullups and pushups hit many muscles, but I really needed more work on my arms and shoulders.

I had always had skinny arms, so my aim was not necessarily to get bigger, but I wanted to make sure I was challenging my body more evenly than I had been up to that point. I investigated exercises that might work and found some cleaning, rowing, and pressing exercises that looked applicable.

There were two observations I had, firstly the single weight made the exercises asymmetrical which felt foreign at first but really helped with focusing on form and core strength, secondly the exercises I chose could often use the legs to start the movement, this helped me adapt to the weight and also bring in extra benefit in my limited routines.

Within a month or two the weight no longer intimidated me, and although I had been sore in a few places with the asymmetrical nature of some of the movements I eventually stopped experiencing any aftereffects. This now becomes a part of my weekly routine where I dedicate an entire round to using kettlebells on the upper body.

In addition to the arm and shoulder exercises I now also use the kettlebell for deadlifts, squats, single leg deadlifts, and lunges for my leg routine on a different day of the week.

# Bosu Ball

Another device I found useful that has become a part of my routine is the Bosu ball. I initially got it to work on balance and to challenge my core, but I soon found a multitude of benefits. For example, I often invert it for pushups which add an extra dimension to a basic exercise. I also use it for squats and combining with the kettlebell it makes 45lb a worthy weight.

With the ball on the top side, I use it for exercises where I plant my foot such as lunges, step ups, and my kicking circuit. It adds extra challenge to abdominal exercises such as crunches, and leg raises. This all enables me to add variety to my routine as well as to take existing exercises and add more into them.

Perfect for my goals of maximizing benefits in a short amount of time.

## Kegel Exercises and Drinking Water

In addition to adding tools to my routine I also looked at my Kegel muscles. When I was younger, I was able to hold my bladder for hours, despite drinking copious quantities of liquid throughout the day. I now found myself infrequently getting up early in the morning to relieve myself, and on days when I had to take a multi hour commute it was often necessary to interrupt my journey.

This was not helped by another change I had started to make, which was to drink more water throughout the day. As a result, I found myself needing to go to the bathroom more, and it started to get annoying. I felt more hydrated, but at one point I was going a couple of times an hour. I knew something had to change and so I decided to work on my Kegel.

At first, I tried hitting those muscles during various movements, adding to my routine even further, but in the end, I found that finding those muscles was much simpler than I imagined. A common trick is to try and hold a urination and identify the muscles you are using. But why stop there?

I began to challenge myself to hold it in when I was about to go. At first three to five seconds, then release, then a few seconds more, and release. Then extending the holding time until
It was 20-30 seconds if needed. As a result of this training, I found my function to be much restored.

## Rest Days and Injuries

The Compact Workout

At the time of completing this book I have been doing regular daily exercise for just over a year. Doing my planned exercises every day was not always practical; life gets in the way. I also knew that sometimes it is good to have a rest or variety in the routine. I found that the best way to maintain consistent and steady progress was to plan.

In my case, on days I worked from home I could usually find 15-20 minutes to exercise and shower by keeping a little space open on my calendar. On these days I would do my more intense workouts involving pull-ups or kettlebells. On days when I was commuting, beyond the walking exercise I may only do my stretching in the evening, or I might only do the first round of exercises. On the weekends I might be away, or I might have a busy schedule and so I would adapt accordingly. This included allowing myself rest days where I relaxed the intensity, but not completely.

One rule I have is that I should try and do the daily exercises at least 5 days a week, because when I had not done them for more than two days I started to lose the feeling of wellness. I also felt the same with my diet, if I started to eat more than one carb heavy meal a day for two days I felt the impact on my wellbeing. Stretching was also the same, after two days of skipping it, my body started to feel in need of rejuvenation.

With the above in mind, I also try to stagger what I am resting. For example, if I skip exercise I still try to stretch and eat healthily, if I eat a big indulgent meal, I try to still do my exercises and stretch, and so on. This allows me to keep a consistent daily thread rather than creating a complete break. At the very least, no matter what else is going on you can hopefully control what you eat, and if you cannot do that, then just skip breakfast entirely.

Planning rest days is only important if you are not already forced to take them on a regular basis, so use your own judgment.

# The results of my compressed workout

| Age | High intensity | Medium | Low | Health (approx.) |
|---|---|---|---|---|
| 18 | 5hrs | 5hrs | 10hrs | Weight 156 lb.<br>BP 120/70<br>HR 60 |
| 22 | 0hrs | 3hrs | 5hrs | Weight 150lb<br>BP 125/75<br>HR 65 |
| 25 | 1hr | 2hrs | 2hrs | Weight 165lb<br>BP 125/75<br>HR 70 |
| 35 | 0hrs | 3hrs | 2hrs | Weight 185lb<br>BP 130/80<br>HR 70 |
| 40 | 3hrs | 3hrs | 3hrs | Weight 175lb<br>BP 135/80<br>HR 60 |
| 45 | 0hrs | 3hrs | 2hrs | Weight 175lb<br>BP 140/85<br>HR 65 |
| 48 | 0.5hrs | 1.5hrs | 3hrs | Weight 160lb<br>BP 100/66<br>HR 60 |

My blood pressure went from 140/80 to 100/66 (although it eventually leveled at 120/75). My body weight dropped fifteen pounds, my waistline reduced, and I was able to wear clothes more comfortably again. I had more energy, more drive, and more focus. I was able to do more with my children, and more around the home. I felt more confident in my everyday interactions, and more comfortable around people. I had changed my life, and I was comfortable with myself, and my increased happiness spread to those around me.

The truth is that my journey is not complete. There is still more to develop, but I have completed my goal of reaching an improved baseline of health and fitness within the confines of my schedule. I am no longer frustrated and feeling helpless, I feel empowered and able to focus on other areas of my life. I have adapted to my current situation and others can too.

# Summary: Lessons Learned in Fitness and Nutrition

After years of trial and error, I have come to understand that the balance between exercise and diet is crucial yet surprisingly nuanced. Here are the core insights that shaped my journey toward a healthier lifestyle:

## The Challenge of Time and Consistency

Time is a luxury that most of us do not have in abundance, and finding ways to squeeze in effective exercise was a constant battle for me. I faced the issue of needing both a warm-up and a workout intense enough to be effective, but with my schedule, I often had time for neither. This led me to explore interval training, specifically Tabata, which provided an intense workout in a condensed time. However, I quickly learned that traditional Tabata was too harsh on my body. This realization led me to customize a 15-minute routine that worked with, not against, my life. These short, timed workouts became a cornerstone of my daily habits, particularly when I linked them with existing routines like showering. Establishing a consistent rhythm of exercise through association and routine was key to overcoming time constraints.

## The Power of Variety in Exercise

I learned the hard way that relying on a few exercises—no matter how effective they seemed initially—was not sustainable. The body needs balance, mobility, and strength across a wide range of muscle groups, especially as we age. My solution was to create a 3-cycle routine that focused on mobility (hips and spine), strength (core and upper body), and conditioning (legs). This structure allowed me to target different muscle groups while keeping workouts varied and engaging. Tools like resistance bands, kettlebells, and a Bosu ball became integral to adding variety and intensity, challenging my muscles in new ways without requiring excessive time or equipment.

## Nutrition: The Missing Piece of the Puzzle

Despite my increased commitment to exercise, I was not seeing the physical results I wanted—particularly when it came to body fat. It took a deeper dive into nutrition for me to realize that exercise alone is not a magic bullet for weight loss. I discovered that controlling sugar intake and managing insulin spikes were far more important than I had once believed. By shifting my focus from "burning off" calories to reducing glucose spikes through diet, I began to see real changes in my body composition. Simple adjustments—like cutting out fruit juices, adding fermented foods to my meals, and balancing carbohydrates with proteins and fats—had a profound impact on my energy levels, waistline, and overall health.

## Flexibility and Stretching: Supporting Long-Term Health

Through trial and error, flexibility and mobility are just as important as strength. After struggling with soreness and tightness, I integrated regular stretching into my routine, drawing on techniques like Makko Ho and yoga. These practices not only alleviated pain but also improved my posture, core stability, and movement quality. Flexibility training became something I could do during quieter moments, such as watching TV or listening to podcasts, making it easy to incorporate into my life without sacrificing workout time.

# The Importance of Rest and Recovery

One of the hardest lessons I learned was the importance of rest. Over-exercising, especially without adequate recovery time, led to burnout and injuries that set me back. By allowing myself to designate rest days, I gave my body the opportunity to heal and come back stronger. I developed a more flexible approach to fitness—on days when I could not manage a full workout, I prioritized lighter activities like stretching or walking. The goal became consistency over perfection, ensuring that I stayed active without overwhelming myself.

# Mindful Progress and Long-Term Gains

The most important lesson of all was learning to balance my expectations with the realities of my life. I no longer chased short-term results or extreme goals. Instead, I focused on making incremental progress that I could sustain over the long haul. This shift in mindset led to improvements not only in my physical health but in my mental and emotional well-being as well. With time, my overall strength, flexibility, and stamina increased significantly, and those small, daily victories began to add up to something far more significant: a healthier, happier, and more resilient me.

In summary, this was about the evolution of my approach to fitness and nutrition. I have moved from trying to fit into a preconceived mold of health to creating a balanced lifestyle that works for me. An approach that values consistency, variety, and patience. And in that, I have found not just fitness but a deeper sense of wellness.

# Key Points to Remember

- Keep your motivation clear.
- Set realistic time and goal expectations.

- Include contingency plans for unexpected schedule changes.
- Do not skip doing anything for more than two days at a time.
- Balance between mobility, flexibility, strength, and endurance.
- Balance across the body.
- Self-monitor and stay mindful during exercise.

## A Note on Aging and Muscles

As we get older, and during extended periods of inactivity, our bodies natural muscle tone and overall capacity diminish, while at the same time we lose flexibility and movement in the joints. Although that may sound straightforward it is important to understand a key difference between a young body and the same body several decades later. If we are inactive when we are young, there is still a good chance that if we start exercising, the foundation is there. In other words, if I start doing popular activities like lifting weights at the age of twenty, provided I am sensible, I should see a high gain to low injury ratio. However, if I were to follow the same methodology when I am older the foundation may have atrophied. Or, to put it another way, it is more likely that I have developed impingement to my movements, weak supporting muscles, and compensation. Even my base level bone density could have deteriorated. This makes the gain to injury ratio degrade significantly.

This means a couple of things:
1) As we get older, we absolutely must exercise, because our non-exercising baseline is lower in comparison to the same baseline when we were younger.
2) We need to spend more time on building stability, flexibility, and mobility when we are older, otherwise injury could ruin our gains.

# Constantly Upscale Your Eating Behaviors

Eating well is paramount, although exercise is key for keeping the connective tissue conditioned and ready for anything, your ability to take control of what you consume is the most powerful action you can take. Always be on the lookout to select a healthier option when eating. The natural items with a lower glycemic index and good amounts of fiber are better for you. However, it may not always be practical to look things up and put numbers in a calculator, here is a chart you can use to upscale your food.

When you go to get a drink, a snack, or a meal, you can make a healthier ranked selection instead of the one you were about to make. For example, if I were about to drink a soda, I might drink kombucha instead. If I were about to have my second kombucha, I might take spring water instead. This is a better approach than forcing yourself to eat a specific diet, just improving the diet over time is enough, and more sustainable.

| 1 | Spring water |
| --- | --- |
| 2 | Filtered water |
| 3 | Kombucha |
| 4 | Tea/coffee (no sugar) |
| 5 | Elixir drinks (low sugar) |
| 6 | Diluted juice drinks with or without vinegar |
| 7 | Small juice/milk |

**Avoid or limit to once a week:**
Sodas (even diet)
Sugary caffeine drinks

Large juices/smoothies
Milk from oat, nut, soy etc.
Alcohol

| 1 | Vegetables bitter green |
| --- | --- |
| 2 | Vegetables low carb |
| 3 | Seeds |
| 4 | Nuts |
| 5 | Fruits |
| 6 | Kefir/plain yogurt |
| 7 | Pickled foods (kimchi, sauerkraut, pickles) |
| 8 | Sashimi |
| 9 | Meat cooked |
| 10 | Vegetable high carb (corn, potatoes, yams etc.) |
| 11 | Other high starch (bread, pasta, potatoes) |
| 12 | Dried processed snack low carbs |
| 13 | Starchy high carb processed snack |
| 14 | Sugary treats, cakes, ice cream etc. |

## The Compound Benefits

If you spend 15 minutes a day exercising that can reach almost two hours of activity a week. If you cycle through alternating workouts and improve your eating and resting behaviors, you can obtain enormous accumulative benefits:

- Stabilize blood pressure.
- Improve your resting heart rate.
- Put your body fat into healthy ranges.
- Make you stronger.
- Make you faster.
- Make you more flexible.
- Give you stamina.
- Improve your gut function.
- Lower your chance of injury.
- Increase your immune system.
- Lower your risks of disease and illness.
- Improve your mental focus.
- Lower your anxiety.
- Improve your self-view and interpersonal relationships.
- Improve your libido.
- Improve your studies/career.
- Increase your independence.

Most importantly it allows you to better sustain yourself with the activities that keep you so busy in the first place. You can get comfortable with a never-ending cycle of exercise, the most important thing to do is adapt to updated information, the current situation, and improvise from there.

## Implementing Your Own Changes

If you are still reading this book, then perhaps you want to try and implement some of these changes into your life. This can be done by reading the remaining sections to:

## The Compact Workout

1. Understand the compact exercise pattern.
2. Learning the key mobility combination.
3. Learning and preparing for the upper body and leg exercises.
4. Understanding the stretching component.
5. Using the sample routines to plan out a weekly pattern of compact workouts.

# The Exercises

## The Exercise Pattern

The circuit pattern uses the following layout:
- The exercises consist of three cycles.
- Each cycle consists of eight rounds of work.
- Each round consists of 23 seconds of work and 7 seconds of rest.
- There are 15 seconds of rest in between each cycle.

# The Compact Workout

| Cycle | Round | Time | Cycle | Round | Time | Cycle | Round | Time |
|---|---|---|---|---|---|---|---|---|
| 1 | 1 | 23s | 2 | 1 | 23s | 3 | 1 | 23s |
| Rest | | 7s | Rest | | 7s | Rest | | 7s |
| 1 | 2 | 23s | 2 | 2 | 23s | 3 | 2 | 23s |
| Rest | | 7s | Rest | | 7s | Rest | | 7s |
| 1 | 3 | 23s | 2 | 3 | 23s | 3 | 3 | 23s |
| Rest | | 7s | Rest | | 7s | Rest | | 7s |
| 1 | 4 | 23s | 2 | 4 | 23s | 3 | 4 | 23s |
| Rest | | 7s | Rest | | 7s | Rest | | 7s |
| 1 | 5 | 23s | 2 | 5 | 23s | 3 | 5 | 23s |
| Rest | | 7s | Rest | | 7s | Rest | | 7s |
| 1 | 6 | 23s | 2 | 6 | 23s | 3 | 6 | 23s |
| Rest | | 7s | Rest | | 7s | Rest | | 7s |
| 1 | 7 | 23s | 2 | 7 | 23s | 3 | 7 | 23s |
| Rest | | 7s | Rest | | 7s | Rest | | 7s |
| 1 | 8 | 23s | 2 | 8 | 23s | 3 | 8 | 23s |
| Rest | | 22s | Rest | | 22s | Total | | 12m 23s |

In the following section I have listed exercises that you can fit into each of these rounds. Usually, I reserve the first eight rounds for my Key Mobility Combination.

# The Key Mobility Combination

This 8-exercise combination should always precede the other activities unless you have a specific reason. If time is limited on a given day, then opt for this combination. If you do not perform them as part of a circuit routine, then timing is not necessary and instead perform nine repetitions of each. If performing as a timed exercise, and once you become familiar with them, there is no need to stop during the rest times and you can simply begin the next exercises as soon as you are ready.

## Cat Cows

Start on all fours, palms down and on the balls of your feet. Focus on large inhales and exhales. As you inhale raise your head up and drop your abdomen relaxing it completely trying to flex the entire length of your spine, while doing so roll your eyes to the top of the sockets, push the tongue to the top of the mouth, and push your knees and palms into the ground and away from each other. As you exhale, drop your head, roll your eyes to the bottom of the sockets and push your tongue into the base of your mouth, round your shoulders, and flex your spine in the opposite direction by contracting your abdomen and chest, while pushing your knees and palms into the floor and towards each other.

Purpose: This exercise fires up the muscles of your spine and hips, increases circulation, coordinates your nervous system, strengthens core and back muscles, and stretches your core, back, hips, and shoulders.

## Alternate Figure Four and Single Leg Bridges

Lie on your back, put your right foot flat on the floor about a foot length down away from your buttocks, put your left foot across the front of the right thigh and keep it flexed. Bring the right foot of the floor as you perform a crunch with your upper body breathing out steadily, then lower the right foot back in place while breathing back in, and drive the right foot into the floor so that your hips rise into the air, as your hips raise into a bridge let the left knee fall away from you stretching the inner thigh while again breathing out. Lower back to the starting position while breathing in and repeat.

As this is asymmetrical exercise you will do two sets, reversing on the second set.

Lie on your back, put your left foot flat on the floor about a foot length down away from your buttocks, put your right foot across the front of the left thigh and keep it flexed. Bring the left foot of the floor as you perform a crunch with your upper body breathing out steadily, then lower the left foot back in place while breathing back in, and drive the left foot into the floor so that your hips rise into the air, as your hips raise into a bridge let the right knee fall away from you stretching the inner thigh while again breathing out. Lower back to the starting position while breathing in and repeat.

Purpose: opens the hips from four different directions, shortens the hamstring to reduce pelvic tilt, engages the core, strengthens the spine, and coordinates the body.

Variations:
Start with just the crunches, using an exercise ball if required, and add a set of double leg bridges elsewhere in the routing until this feels more comfortable.


## Floor Spine Rotations with Shoulder Discipline

Still lying on your back, bring your elbows up level with your shoulders on the floor, if possible, bend your elbows and put the back of your hands on the floor above the elbows so that your arms are bent at 90 degrees. Raise your knees so that they are above the line of your waist, with the knees bent to 90 degrees. Turn your head to look to the right and lower your knees to the left without letting your shoulders or hands lose contact with the floor, slowly and smoothly alternate to the other side. Repeat this exercise until the round time is complete, but do not rush it, instead "hang out" in the extended position without creating discomfort. Breathe naturally.

Purpose: Wrings out the spine, promotes sacral flexibility, stretches the outside of the hip, unlocks the lumbar vertebrae by loosening the muscles of the low back, supports and mobilizes the neck, encourages alignment of the shoulders.

Variations: use an exercise ball to raise the legs, put the arms palm down out to the sides for support. If this is also too challenging, leave your feet on the floor and simply bring your knees from side to side.

## Asian Squat Upper Spine Rotations with Chest/Shoulder Stretch

From a flat-footed deep squat rest your elbows inside your knees. Bring the right arm around behind and extend the hand outwards and upwards while also turning the head and looking at the extended hand. Breathe in while extending. The left arm and elbow braces on the left leg for support. Return to the starting position with an exhale and repeat on the other side.

Purpose: Stretches the glutes, calves, and tendons of the knee. Encourages mobility in the thoracic vertebrae, further loosens the neck.

Variations: This exercise can also be performed from a kneeling position or on all fours.

## Extended Front Leg Thread the Needle and Outer Rotations

From a right lunge position with the rear foot active, extend the right foot as far forward as possible while leaving a little room between the right thigh and the floor. Put the right hand to the left of the right foot then reach your left hand as deep as you can under the right thigh while also bringing your head in the same direction and rotating your spine to the right to look under your right leg. Breathe out to relieve abdominal pressure. You may also opt to slightly straighten the right knee to allow a deeper twist of the hips.

Return through the starting position and while keeping the right hand on the floor extend the left hand up and out behind you while following your hand with your gaze and taking a deep inhale. You may opt to slightly bend the knee to facilitate the opening of the hips.

Purpose: Engage and maintain core, shoulder/hip/spine/neck rotation.

## 50/50 with CAR Shoulder Rotations to Pigeon Pose

In this exercise, you start by sitting on the floor with your knees bent and feet positioned wider than hip-width apart. While leaning back slightly for support, you drop both knees to the right side, letting them fall toward the floor. This motion allows one leg to internally rotate while the other externally rotates, stretching and mobilizing the hips. As you bring the knees to the floor then raise the left hand up in a wide arc. Roll your body over the right hip and extend the left leg behind you and fold at the waist while extending both hands in front of you.

You then return the knees to the center and repeat the movement on the opposite side, alternating in a controlled manner. Keeping your torso upright as much as possible is key to ensuring the hips are the focus of the stretch, rather than compensating with the lower back.

Purpose: Improves hip flexibility and range of motion. Increasing the mobility, strength, and overall function of the shoulder joint. Stretches the hip flexors, glutes, and piriformis.

# Upper Body and Core Exercises

I usually choose my next eight rounds from this section of exercises, although I may also repeat the same exercise up to three times in the same cycle depending on my goals that week.

## Floor Work

These are exercises that require only a flat surface.

### Push Ups

Lie on your front, put your palms vertically on the floor with your fingertips in line with your nipples, and your elbows close to the sides of your body. Engage your core, pinch your shoulders together at the back and push up, until your arms are almost fully extended. Then slowly lower yourself back to the floor.

Alternatively perform this exercise by keeping your knees on the floor.

### Archer Push Ups

The archer pushup is a challenging variation of the standard pushup that shifts most of the body weight to one arm, targeting the chest, shoulders, and triceps while enhancing stability and core strength. Start in a plank position with your hands wider than shoulder-width apart. As you lower your body, focus on one arm while keeping the other extended straight out to the side.

Lower yourself towards the ground by bending the elbow of the working arm, keeping the opposite arm straight throughout. Push back up, then alternate sides or complete all reps on one side before switching. This exercise builds unilateral strength and serves as a progression towards one-arm pushups.

## Pike Push Ups

A pike pushup is a bodyweight exercise that primarily targets the shoulders, triceps, and upper chest while also engaging the core. To perform it, start in a downward dog position with your hips elevated and your body forming an inverted V-shape. Your hands should be shoulder-width apart, and your feet should be close together.

From this position, lower your head towards the floor by bending your elbows, mimicking a vertical pressing motion. Once your head is close to the ground, push through your hands to return to the starting position. Pike push-ups are excellent for building shoulder strength and can be a progression towards handstand pushups.

## V-Ups

A V-up is a core exercise that targets the abdominal muscles, especially the rectus abdominis, while also engaging the hip flexors. Start by lying flat on your back with your arms extended overhead and legs straight. Simultaneously lift your arms and legs off the ground, bringing them towards each other to form a "V" shape with your body.

At the top of the movement, your hands should meet your feet, with your upper and lower body elevated off the ground. Slowly lower back down to the starting position, keeping control throughout the movement. V-ups are excellent for improving core strength and stability while also challenging your balance and coordination.

## Crunches

A crunch is a simple and effective core exercise that primarily targets the upper abdominal muscles. To perform it, start by lying on your back with your knees bent and feet flat on the ground. Place your hands behind your head or across over your chest for support.

Engage your core to lift your shoulders and upper back off the ground while keeping your lower back in contact with the floor. At the top of the movement, squeeze your abdominal muscles, then slowly lower back down. Crunches help improve core strength and definition by focusing on the upper portion of the abdominal muscles.

## Flutter Kicks

Flutter kicks are a core exercise that targets the lower abdominal muscles and hip flexors while also engaging the quads. To perform them, lie flat on your back with your legs extended and your arms resting at your sides or tucked under your hips for support. Lift both legs a few inches off the ground and begin alternating kicks, raising one leg while lowering the other in a controlled, continuous motion.

Keep your core engaged throughout the movement, maintaining a steady pace without letting your legs touch the floor. Flutter kicks help improve lower abdominal strength and endurance, while also enhancing overall core stability.

## Superman Plank

A Superman Plank is a dynamic core exercise that challenges your stability while engaging multiple muscle groups, particularly the core, shoulders, and glutes. Begin in a high plank position with your hands placed under your shoulders and your body in a straight line from head to toe. From this position, lift one arm straight out in front of you while simultaneously lifting the opposite leg off the ground, maintaining balance and control.

Hold this position briefly, then return to the plank and repeat on the opposite side. This exercise not only strengthens the core but also improves balance, coordination, and full-body stability, making it an excellent alternative to the traditional Superman exercise. The alternating arm and leg lifts add an additional challenge to your core as it works to keep your body steady throughout the movement.

## Handstands

A handstand is a fundamental gymnastic and bodyweight exercise that primarily targets the shoulders, arms, and core, while also enhancing balance and coordination. To perform a handstand, begin in a standing position with your arms raised overhead. Lean forward into a lunge and place your hands shoulder-width apart on the ground, then kick your legs up into the air until your body is fully inverted. Engage your core and squeeze your glutes to maintain a straight, vertical line from head to toe.

Hold the handstand position by balancing on your hands, using your core and shoulders to stabilize. To exit, slowly lower your legs back to the ground in a controlled motion. Handstands are excellent for building upper body strength, particularly in the shoulders, and improving overall body control and balance. This exercise should utilize wall support for beginners, eventually progressing to freestanding handstands as strength and stability increase.

## Bands

These exercises require a looped exercise band of adequate length and resistance.

### Arm Curls

Arm curls with an exercise band are a wonderful way to target the biceps while also engaging the stabilizer muscles in your arms and core. To perform the exercise, start by standing on the middle of the band with your feet shoulder-width apart. Hold the handles or ends of the band in both hands, palms facing forward, and let your arms hang by your sides.

Keeping your elbows close to your torso, curl both hands upwards simultaneously by contracting your biceps. Continue the motion until your hands reach shoulder height, then slowly lower them back to the starting position with control. Exercise band arm curls provide resistance through the entire range of motion, making them a highly effective bicep-building exercise that can be performed anywhere.

### Upright Rows

Upright rows with an exercise band effectively target the shoulders, traps, and upper back. To perform this exercise, stand on the middle of the band with your feet shoulder-width apart, holding the handles or ends of the band in both hands with your palms facing your thighs and your hands close together in front of you.

Pull the band upwards by raising your elbows, keeping the handles close to your body. Continue lifting until your elbows are at shoulder height and your hands are just under your chin. Hold for a moment, then slowly lower your hands back to the starting position. This exercise is excellent for building shoulder and upper back strength while using the resistance of the band to engage stabilizer muscles throughout the movement.

## Shoulder Press

A band shoulder press is a powerful exercise for building shoulder strength while also engaging the triceps and upper chest. To perform this exercise, stand on the middle of the band with your feet shoulder-width apart. Hold the handles or ends of the band at shoulder height with your palms facing forward and your elbows bent at about 90 degrees.

Press the band upward by extending your arms overhead until they are fully extended, keeping your core engaged and maintaining a straight back. Once your arms are fully extended, pause briefly at the top, then slowly lower the handles back down to shoulder height with control. The band shoulder press effectively strengthens the shoulders while allowing for smooth, adjustable resistance throughout the movement, making it an excellent alternative to using free weights.

## Band Pull-apart

The band pull-apart is an excellent exercise for strengthening the upper back, shoulders, and rear deltoids, as well as improving posture and shoulder stability. Begin by standing with your feet shoulder-width apart and holding an exercise band in front of you at shoulder height, with your arms extended and hands slightly wider than shoulder-width. The band should have light tension at the start. Keeping your arms straight (but not locked), pull the band apart by drawing your hands outward and slightly down until your arms align with your sides, focusing on squeezing your shoulder blades together as you complete the movement.

Hold the peak position briefly to fully engage the upper back muscles, then slowly return your arms to the starting position with control, maintaining tension in the band. Band pull-aparts are an effective way to strengthen the muscles that support good posture and shoulder alignment, particularly the rhomboids and rear deltoids. This exercise is also frequently recommended as a corrective movement to balance out the effects of a forward-slump posture or excessive pressing movements.

## Push Ups with Band

Band-assisted push-ups are an excellent way to add resistance to the traditional pushup, increasing the challenge to the chest, shoulders, and triceps while also engaging the core. To perform a pushup with a band, begin by looping the band around your upper back, holding the ends in your hands. Position yourself in a pushup position with your hands slightly wider than shoulder-width apart and the band secured under your palms. Your body should be in a straight line from head to toe.

As you lower your body towards the ground, the resistance of the band increases the intensity of the movement, forcing your muscles to work harder as you push back up. Once you reach the bottom of the pushup, press back up through your palms against the band's resistance to return to the starting position. This exercise is great for building strength and endurance in the upper body while offering a progressive challenge as the band adds consistent resistance throughout the range of motion.

# Kettlebells

## Single Arm Bicep Cleans

The single-arm kettlebell clean is a powerful movement that targets the posterior chain, shoulders, and core while building explosive strength and coordination. To perform the exercise, start with the kettlebell on the ground between your feet, with your feet shoulder-width apart. Hinge at your hips, keeping your back straight, and grab the kettlebell with one hand. In one explosive motion, extend your hips and knees to generate power, pulling the kettlebell up towards your shoulder. As the kettlebell rises, rotate your wrist so that the kettlebell smoothly transitions to rest against your forearm, ending in a rack position with the kettlebell at shoulder height.

Once the kettlebell is in the rack position, stand tall, squeezing your glutes and core for stability. To reset, lower the kettlebell back down to the starting position with control, ensuring your back remains straight throughout the movement. The single-arm kettlebell clean is a versatile exercise that not only builds strength but also enhances grip, coordination, and overall body control, making it a key component in functional training routines.

## Double Handed Shoulder Press

A double-handed kettlebell shoulder press is an excellent upper body strength exercise that primarily targets the shoulders while also engaging the triceps, upper chest, and core for stability. To perform the exercise, stand with your feet shoulder-width apart and hold the kettlebell with both hands by the handle, starting at chest height. Your elbows should be bent and close to your body. Engage your core and glutes to maintain a solid base.

From this position, press the kettlebell upward in a controlled motion, fully extending your arms overhead while keeping your wrists neutral and avoiding any arching of your lower back. Once you reach the top, pause briefly before slowly lowering the kettlebell back down to the starting position at chest height. The double-handed kettlebell shoulder press is a fantastic way to develop shoulder strength and stability while ensuring that the core is actively engaged throughout the movement to support proper form.

## Single Handed Shoulder Press

A single-handed kettlebell shoulder press is an excellent exercise for building unilateral shoulder strength, stability, and coordination, while also engaging the core for balance. To perform the exercise, start by holding a kettlebell in one hand at shoulder height, with your palm facing forward and the kettlebell resting against the back of your forearm in a rack position. Stand with your feet shoulder-width apart, engaging your core and glutes to maintain stability.

From this position, press the kettlebell overhead in a controlled motion, extending your arm fully without allowing your body to sway or your lower back to arch. Once your arm is fully extended overhead, pause briefly before slowly lowering the kettlebell back to the starting position at shoulder height. The single-handed kettlebell shoulder press effectively develops shoulder strength and stability while promoting balance and coordination due to the unilateral nature of the exercise, making it a key movement in functional strength training routines.

## Single Arm Bent Rows

The single-arm kettlebell bent row is a powerful exercise that targets the upper back, lats, and biceps while also engaging the core to maintain stability. To perform this exercise, start by standing with your feet shoulder-width apart and a slight bend in your knees. Hinge at the hips, keeping your back straight, and grip the kettlebell with one hand while the other hand can rest on your knee or a stable surface for support. Your torso should be almost parallel to the ground.

From this position, pull the kettlebell towards your ribcage by driving your elbow upwards while keeping it close to your body. Squeeze your shoulder blade at the top of the movement, then slowly lower the kettlebell back to the starting position with control. The single arm bent row is excellent for strengthening the upper back muscles and improving posture, while also helping to correct muscle imbalances by training one side at a time.

## Upright Two-Handed Rows

The two-handed kettlebell upright row is a great exercise for targeting the shoulders, traps, and upper back while also engaging the biceps. To perform the exercise, stand with your feet shoulder-width apart and hold the kettlebell with both hands in front of your body, palms facing your thighs. Your arms should be straight, and the kettlebell should be hanging down.

From this starting position, pull the kettlebell upwards towards your chin, leading with your elbows. Your elbows should flare out to the sides as you lift, and the kettlebell should stay close to your body. Continue pulling until your elbows are at shoulder height and the kettlebell is just below your chin. Pause briefly at the top, then slowly lower the kettlebell back down to the starting position with control. The two-handed kettlebell upright row is an effective movement for building strength in the shoulders and traps while also improving posture and upper body stability.

## Kneeling Halos

Kneeling kettlebell halos are a variation of the traditional halo exercise that further emphasizes core engagement and shoulder stability by reducing the base of support. To perform kneeling halos, start by kneeling on the ground with your knees hip-width apart and your body upright. Hold the kettlebell by the horns in front of your chest, with your elbows bent and the bell part hanging down.

From this position, initiate the halo by slowly rotating the kettlebell around your head, moving it over one shoulder, behind your head, and over the other shoulder, bringing it back to the starting position in front of your chest. As with the standing version, keep your head still and engage your core to prevent your torso from twisting during the movement. After completing the desired number of rotations in one direction, reverse the movement and repeat in the opposite direction. Kneeling halos not only improve shoulder mobility and strength but also require greater balance and core stabilization due to the kneeling posture, making them excellent all-around upper body exercise.

## Side Bends

Kettlebell side bends are a simple yet effective exercise for targeting the obliques, the muscles along the sides of your core, while also engaging the lower back and hips. To perform the exercise, stand with your feet shoulder-width apart and hold a kettlebell in one hand at your side. Keep your back straight and your core engaged as you slowly bend sideways at the waist, lowering the kettlebell towards the ground. Make sure to keep the movement controlled, avoiding any twisting or leaning forward.

Once you have reached a comfortable stretch in your obliques, use those muscles to pull your torso back up to the starting position. Repeat for the desired number of reps, then switch the kettlebell to the other hand and perform the exercise on the opposite side. Kettlebell side bends help improve core strength and stability, specifically focusing on the lateral muscles, while also helping to increase flexibility and balance in your torso.

## Pullup Bar

## Pullups (with band)

A band-assisted pull-up is an effective way to build the strength needed for full, unassisted pull-ups. To perform the exercise, loop a resistance band securely around a pull-up bar. Place one or both feet (or knees) into the band, depending on how much assistance you need. The thicker the band, the more assistance it provides. Grip the bar with your palms facing away (overhand) or towards you (underhand), slightly wider than shoulder-width apart.

From this position, engage your core and pull yourself upward, leading with your chest and keeping your shoulders down and back. As you pull, the band will assist you by providing upward momentum, making it easier to lift your body weight. Once your chin clears the bar, pause briefly before lowering yourself back down in a controlled manner to the starting position. Band-assisted pull-ups are a terrific way to improve upper body strength and work towards unassisted pull-ups by gradually using less assistance over time.

## Pullups

A regular pull-up is a fundamental bodyweight exercise that primarily targets the upper body, particularly the back (latissimus dorsi), shoulders, biceps, and core. To perform a pull-up, begin by gripping a pull-up bar with your palms facing away from you (overhand grip), slightly wider than shoulder-width apart. Hang from the bar with your arms fully extended and your body in a straight line.

Engage your core and back muscles as you pull yourself upward, leading with your chest and drawing your elbows down and back. Continue pulling until your chin clears the bar. Pause briefly at the top, then slowly lower yourself back down in a controlled manner to the starting position with your arms fully extended. Regular pull-ups are a fantastic exercise for building upper body strength, improving grip, and developing muscle endurance in the back and arms.

## Chin Ups (with Band)

A band-assisted chin-up is a wonderful way to build strength for full chin-ups, targeting the biceps, shoulders, and back muscles. To perform this exercise, start by securely looping a resistance band around a pull-up bar. Place one or both feet (or knees) into the band, depending on how much assistance you need. Grip the bar with your palms facing towards you (underhand grip), about shoulder-width apart.

From this starting position, engage your core and pull your body upward by bending your elbows and drawing them down towards your sides. The band will assist in providing upward momentum, reducing the amount of body weight you are lifting. Continue pulling until your chin clears the bar. Pause briefly at the top, then lower yourself back down in a controlled manner to the starting position. Band-assisted chin-ups are ideal for those working towards unassisted chin-ups by gradually reducing band assistance as strength improves.

## Chin-ups

A regular chin-up is a bodyweight exercise that focuses on building upper body strength, particularly in the biceps, shoulders, and back muscles. To perform a chin-up, start by gripping a pull-up bar with an underhand grip (palms facing towards you), shoulder-width apart. Hang from the bar with your arms fully extended and your body in a straight line.

Engage your core and begin the movement by pulling your body upward, driving your elbows down and squeezing your biceps. Continue pulling until your chin clears the bar. Once at the top, pause briefly before lowering yourself back down in a controlled manner until your arms are fully extended again. Regular chin-ups are excellent for building bicep strength while also engaging the back, making them an effective exercise for overall upper body development.

## Bosu Ball

### Bosu Push Ups

Bosu ball push-ups with the flat side facing up are an even more advanced variation that significantly enhances core engagement, balance, and upper body strength. To perform this exercise, place the Bosu ball on the ground with the flat side up. Grip the edges of the flat platform with both hands and position your body in a pushup position, keeping your hands slightly wider than shoulder-width apart. Your body should form a straight line from head to toe, with your feet together or hip-width apart for stability.

Lower your chest towards the Bosu ball by bending your elbows, maintaining a controlled movement to avoid tipping the ball. Keep your core tight to help stabilize your body. Once your chest is near the Bosu ball, push through your palms to return to the starting position. The flat side up creates a highly unstable surface, forcing your core, shoulders, and stabilizer muscles to work harder to maintain balance throughout the movement, making it a challenging variation that improves strength, stability, and overall coordination.

## Bosu Balance Crunch

Bosu ball crunches are an effective exercise for targeting the abdominal muscles while also engaging the core stabilizers due to the unstable surface. To perform a Bosu ball crunch, place the Bosu ball on the floor with the dome side up. Sit on the ball with your lower back resting against the dome, ensuring that your hips are slightly forward. Your feet should be flat on the ground, about hip-width apart, and your knees bent.

Lean back slightly, allowing the curve of the Bosu ball to support your lower back. Place your hands behind your head or across your chest for support. Engage your core, then lift your upper body towards your knees in a crunching motion. As you curl up, focus on contracting your abdominal muscles and keep your lower back in contact with the ball. Once you reach the top of the movement, slowly lower yourself back down to the starting position. Bosu ball crunches increase the challenge compared to traditional crunches by forcing your stabilizer muscles to work harder, enhancing core strength and balance.

## Cross Crunches

The Bosu Ball Cross Crunch is a core-focused exercise that engages your abdominal muscles, particularly the obliques, while challenging your balance and coordination. To perform the exercise, position the Bosu ball dome side up on the floor and lie on your back with your lower back resting on the dome. Extend your legs out in front of you and keep your arms extended to the sides for stability. Begin the movement by raising one leg and simultaneously reaching across your body with the opposite arm, performing a cross-body crunch. Focus on rotating your torso and engaging your obliques as you reach for the opposite foot.

Once you have reached towards your leg, return to the starting position with control and repeat on the other side. The alternating movement works to tone the oblique muscles while also enhancing core stability and flexibility. The instability of the Bosu ball adds an extra challenge to the exercise, forcing your body to stabilize as you move, which improves balance and engages the deeper core muscles. This exercise is effective for building core strength and improving overall coordination.

## Leg Exercises

I usually reserve the last eight rounds for leg exercises, and due to my interest in martial arts I tend to do a lot of kicking exercises each week. I find these good for overall hip stability, and functional in my other training. You may choose other leg exercises that suit you better.

## Assisted Front Stamp Kick

Performing a front stamp kick with assistance allows you to maintain balance and focus on proper form, making it ideal for beginners or those building strength. To perform the assisted front stamp kick, stand next to a stable object like a wall, chair, or barre, and lightly hold onto it with one hand for support. Start with your feet shoulder-width apart and bring your hands into a guard position, with one hand remaining on the stable object.

Shift your weight onto one leg while lifting the opposite knee toward your chest in preparation for the kick. Extend your leg forward in a controlled, stamping motion, pushing through your heel as if stamping onto a target in front of you. Flex your foot and focus on maintaining control through your core. After the leg is fully extended, hold briefly before retracting it and lowering it back to the starting position. Perform the desired number of reps before switching to the other leg. Using assistance ensures stability, allowing you to refine your kicking technique while safely building lower body strength and coordination.

## Assisted Back Stamp Kick

To perform an assisted back stamp kick, stand facing a stable object such as a chair, wall, or barre, lightly holding onto it for balance. Start with your feet shoulder-width apart and engage your core to maintain stability. As you prepare to kick, shift your weight onto the base leg, slightly bending that knee for balance. Hinge forward at the hip on your base leg, keeping your back flat and your chest up. This hinge will allow your kicking leg to extend higher without compromising your form.

Lift your opposite knee towards your chest, then extend it back in a controlled, stamping motion. Push through the heel as you kick backwards, aiming for height without arching your lower back or leaning excessively forward. The hinging motion helps maximize the range of motion in your kick by allowing your leg to travel higher while maintaining proper posture and core engagement. After fully extending your leg, pause briefly before retracting it and returning to the starting position. Repeat the desired number of reps before switching to the other leg. This technique, combined with assistance for balance, ensures you can focus on precision, strength, and flexibility in your back stamp kick.

## Assisted Side Kick

Lunge squats are a combination of lunges and squats that work to build strength in the lower body, particularly targeting the quadriceps, hamstrings, glutes, and calves. To perform a lunge squat, start by standing tall with your feet hip-width apart and your hands on your hips or by your sides. Step forward with one leg into a lunge position by bending both knees until your back knee is close to the ground and your front knee is directly above your ankle. From this position, lower your hips into a squat by bending both knees further into the lunge, then push through the heel of your front foot to return to the standing position. Repeat on the other leg to complete one rep.

You can also perform lunge squats by stepping backwards instead of forwards. Begin in the same standing position with feet hip-width apart. Step one leg back into a reverse lunge, lowering your back knee towards the floor and bending your front knee over your ankle. Drop your hips into a squat position at the lowest point of the lunge, then press through your front heel to rise back to the standing position. Alternating between stepping forward and stepping backward in your lunge squats helps to engage different muscle groups while enhancing balance and coordination, making this a powerful lower body exercise.

## Squats

The free-standing squat is a fundamental bodyweight exercise that primarily targets the quadriceps, hamstrings, glutes, and core, while also promoting mobility and stability in the lower body. To perform a free-standing squat, begin by standing tall with your feet shoulder-width apart and your toes pointing slightly outward. Engage your core to stabilize your torso, and keep your chest lifted as you initiate the movement by pushing your hips back, as if you are sitting down into a chair. As you lower yourself, bend your knees while keeping them aligned over your toes, aiming to lower your thighs until they are parallel to the ground, or as low as your mobility allows.

At the bottom of the squat, ensure that your weight is distributed evenly through your heels, not the toes, to avoid unnecessary strain on your knees. Once you reach the lowest point of your squat, press through your heels to push yourself back up to the starting position, fully extending your hips and knees at the top. Free-standing squats are excellent for building lower body strength and improving functional movement, as they mimic everyday motions like sitting and standing. They also help to increase flexibility in the hips and ankles, while engaging the core muscles for stability and balance throughout the movement.

## The Bosu Ball Squat (also with Kettlebell)

The Bosu ball squat with the dome side down enhances core stability, balance, and lower body strength. To perform this exercise, start by flipping the Bosu ball so that the flat side is facing up and the dome side is down on the floor. Stand carefully on the flat surface, positioning your feet shoulder-width apart. Engage your core for stability, and make sure your body is upright before you begin. As with any squat, start by pushing your hips back as if sitting in a chair, and begin to bend your knees.

As you lower into the squat, focus on keeping your balance on the unstable surface. Your knees should track over your toes, and your chest should remain lifted. Lower yourself until your thighs are parallel to the ground (or as low as your stability allows), then push through your heels to rise back up to the standing position. The instability of the Bosu ball forces the muscles in your legs, core, and ankles to work harder to maintain balance throughout the movement, making this variation of the squat particularly effective for improving functional strength, proprioception, and coordination.

## Lunge Squat (can also be done with kettlebell)

Lunge squats are a combination of lunges and squats that work to build strength in the lower body, particularly targeting the quadriceps, hamstrings, glutes, and calves. To perform a lunge squat, start by standing tall with your feet hip-width apart and your hands on your hips or by your sides. Step forward with one leg into a lunge position by bending both knees until your back knee is close to the ground and your front knee is directly above your ankle. From this position, lower your hips into a squat by bending both knees further into the lunge, then push through the heel of your front foot to return to the standing position. Repeat on the other leg to complete one rep.

You can also perform lunge squats by stepping backwards instead of forwards. Begin in the same standing position with feet hip-width apart. Step one leg back into a reverse lunge, lowering your back knee towards the floor and bending your front knee over your ankle. Drop your hips into a squat position at the lowest point of the lunge, then press through your front heel to rise back to the standing position. Alternating between stepping forward and stepping backward in your lunge squats helps to engage different muscle groups while enhancing balance and coordination, making this a powerful lower body exercise.

## Single Leg Box Squat

The single-leg box squat is a powerful unilateral exercise that strengthens the quadriceps, hamstrings, glutes, and core while also enhancing balance and stability. To perform the exercise, stand beside a sturdy box or chair and place one foot on the elevated surface with the leg extended straight and relaxed. The other leg remains firmly on the ground, and you will squat with this leg. Engage your core to maintain stability and, while keeping your chest upright, hinge slightly at the hips. Begin lowering your body by bending the knee of the standing leg, slowly squatting towards the floor while keeping the elevated leg straight and passive.

As you lower yourself into the squat, maintain control by focusing on balance and ensuring your knee tracks over your toes. Once you reach a comfortable depth (or just before your other leg touches the ground), push through the heel of your standing leg to return to the starting position. This exercise effectively builds lower body strength while challenging your balance and coordination due to its unilateral nature. It is a fantastic way to improve stability in each leg independently and correct muscle imbalances.

## Bosu Ball Squats

Performing squats on a Bosu ball with the flat side up is a more challenging variation of the traditional squat that enhances balance, stability, and core engagement. To perform this exercise, place the Bosu ball on the ground with the flat side up and carefully step onto the center of the dome, positioning your feet about shoulder-width apart. Engage your core and maintain an upright posture as you begin the squat by pushing your hips back and lowering your body as you would in a regular squat. Keep your weight centered over the Bosu ball and lower yourself until your thighs are parallel to the floor (or as low as is comfortable), ensuring that your knees are aligned with your toes.

Once at the bottom of the squat, press through your heels to return to the standing position, fully extending your hips and knees at the top. The unstable surface of the Bosu ball forces your core, ankles, and stabilizer muscles to work harder to maintain balance throughout the movement, making this variation excellent for improving functional strength, coordination, and lower body endurance. Squats on the Bosu ball are particularly beneficial for athletes or individuals looking to enhance balance and proprioception.

## Bosu Ball Step Ups with Knee Raises

Step-ups on a Bosu ball with a knee raise are a more dynamic variation of the traditional step-up, further challenging balance and coordination while engaging the core, glutes, quadriceps, and hamstrings. To perform this exercise, place the Bosu ball dome-side up on the ground and stand facing it with your feet about hip-width apart. Engage your core and keep your posture upright throughout the movement.

Step one foot onto the center of the Bosu ball, ensuring stability. Push through the heel of the foot on the Bosu ball to lift your body up, while simultaneously driving the opposite knee upwards towards your chest into a knee raise. Hold the knee raise briefly at the top to enhance core activation, then lower the raised leg back down to the ground in a controlled motion, followed by stepping off the Bosu ball with the lead foot. Alternate legs and repeat the movement. Adding the knee raise intensifies the exercise by challenging balance further and increasing engagement of the core and hip flexors.

## Wall Ankle Mobility Drill

The Wall Ankle Mobility Drill is an effective exercise designed to improve ankle dorsiflexion, a crucial movement for activities such as squatting, running, and jumping. To perform the exercise, stand facing a wall with one foot positioned a few inches away from the base, toes pointing forward. Engage your core and ensure your heel is planted firmly on the ground throughout the movement. Slowly push your knee forward towards the wall, aiming to touch it without lifting your heel. It is important to keep the ankle straight during this movement to properly target the ankle joint and surrounding muscles.

Once your knee either touches the wall or reaches its maximum forward range without the heel lifting, pause for a brief stretch, then return to the starting position. Repeat this motion for several reps before switching to the other leg. The wall ankle mobility drill helps increase flexibility and mobility in the ankle joint, which can reduce the risk of injury and improve performance in lower-body exercises that require deep ankle flexion, such as squats and lunges. It is particularly useful for athletes, individuals recovering from ankle injuries, or anyone seeking to improve their range of motion.

# Stretching

## Warm Up

To warm up for stretching I do thirty each leg of the following:
- Forward and backward leg swings
- Sideways leg swings toes forward
- Sideways leg swings toes upward

## Box Split

To perform a side split, start by standing with your feet together, then step out to the side with one leg while keeping the other leg straight, allowing your hips to open as you lower your body toward the floor. Gradually slide your legs apart, using your hands for support on the ground or against a wall to maintain balance and control. Focus on keeping your hips square and your back straight as you lower yourself, aiming to reach a comfortable depth without forcing the stretch. Hold the position while breathing deeply, and then carefully return to the starting position. I practice the box split sitting on a small chair so that I can rest into the stretch, holding for 30-60 seconds over two rounds, alternating with the front splits.

## Front Split

To perform a front split, begin by standing with your feet together, then step one foot forward into a lunge position, bending that knee while keeping the other leg straight behind you. Gradually lower your hips down, sliding your front foot forward and your back foot back, while maintaining a straight back and keeping your hips square. Use your hands for balance on the ground if needed and focus on relaxing into the stretch without forcing it. Aim to reach a comfortable depth, holding the position while breathing deeply, and then carefully return to the starting position. I again use a small chair for side support, with the focus on stretching the front thigh of the back leg by keeping the core upright. While alternating my position into the side split, I pay careful attention to release the pressure as I move.

## Butterfly Stretch

To perform a butterfly stretch, sit on the floor with your back straight and your feet together, allowing your knees to drop out to the sides. Grasp your feet with both hands and gently pull them closer to your body, keeping your spine tall. From this position, slowly lean forward at the hips while maintaining a straight back, aiming to bring your chest toward the floor. Hold the stretch for 20-30 seconds, breathing deeply and relaxing your inner thighs as you deepen the stretch. To release, slowly rise back to an upright position, and repeat as needed to enhance flexibility.

## Forward Fold

To perform a seated forward fold stretch, begin by sitting on the floor with your legs extended straight in front of you. Keep your spine tall, feet flexed, and engage your core. Inhale deeply, then exhale as you hinge forward from the hips, reaching your arms towards your feet. If possible, hold your feet or ankles, but avoid rounding your back. Relax your neck and let your head drop naturally as you breathe deeply, aiming to lengthen the spine with each inhale and fold deeper with each exhale. Hold the stretch for 30 seconds to a minute, focusing on relaxing into the stretch rather than pushing beyond your limits.

## Straddle Stretch

To perform a straddle stretch (pancake stretch), sit on the floor with your legs extended wide in a V shape. Keep your toes flexed and legs straight, pressing your thighs into the ground. Engage your core and sit tall, lengthening your spine. Inhale deeply, then exhale as you hinge forward from the hips, reaching your hands out in front of you, aiming to lower your chest towards the floor. Avoid rounding your back, keeping the movement in your hips. You can support yourself with your hands or elbows, and gradually deepen the stretch with each exhale. Hold the position for 30 seconds to a minute, focusing on steady, deep breaths.

## Reclined Hero Pose

To perform this pose, begin in a kneeling position with your knees together and feet alongside your hips, letting your seat reach the floor between your ankles if your flexibility allows. Slowly lean back, supporting yourself with your hands first, then your elbows, and eventually lying down fully on your back if your flexibility allows. Keep your knees and thighs grounded, and if needed, use props like a bolster or blanket under your back or shoulders for support. Relax your arms by your sides, palms facing upward, and breathe deeply. This pose provides a deep stretch for the thighs and opens the hips while promoting relaxation. Hold the pose for up to a minute, ensuring no discomfort in your lower back or knees.

## Seated Spine Twists

To perform a seated spine twist, sit on the floor with your legs extended straight in front of you. Bend your right knee and cross your right foot over your left thigh, placing it flat on the floor. Keep your left leg extended or bend it, bringing your left foot close to your right hip for a deeper stretch. Inhale and sit tall, lengthening your spine. Exhale as you twist your torso to the right, placing your right hand behind you for support and your left elbow on the outside of your right knee to deepen the twist. Keep your spine long and gaze over your right shoulder, using each inhale to lengthen the spine and each exhale to twist deeper. Hold for 30 seconds to a minute, then switch sides.

## Half Lotus Pose

To perform this stretch, begin by sitting in a comfortable cross-legged position. Then, lift your right foot and place the heel on top of your left thigh, close to the hip crease, with the sole of your foot facing upward. Your left leg remains bent underneath. Sit tall with a straight spine, and keep your shoulders relaxed. If this feels comfortable, you can hold the pose for 30 seconds to a minute, then switch sides by placing your left heel on your right thigh.

# Sample Routines

Here is a typical week that I have followed to implement and sustain the principles described in the book. It is not by any means a large commitment, and that is the entire point of this book. A little bit, for the right person, and the right reason, can go a long way. I change my routine constantly depending on the kind of week I am having as I balance family, work, and other commitments, and I encourage anyone else to develop this flexible mindset. Note also that these are just for reference, and you are free to adapt, or completely overhaul the routines below. It all comes down to what is appropriate for you.

You will see that I have labeled each routine with a named theme to help maintain the broad aspects of the program, and to incorporate flexibility to account for distinct types of days. Exercises repeated in a section indicate multiple sets of the same exercise.

# Day1 - Strict Day

Ideally each week at least one day should be highly dedicated to your healthy lifestyle change, pick the day that is most likely to allow for this.

| | |
|---|---|
| Breakfast | Egg, Kefir & Berries. Coffee |
| Key mobility exercises | All |
| Upper body and core | V ups<br>Crunch<br>Flutter kicks<br>Supermans<br>Bands (curl, rows, press, push-ups) |
| Lower body | Front/back kicks<br>Side kicks<br>Lunge squats<br>Ankle mobility drill |
| Lunch | Tomato, cucumber, olives, feta cheese. Kombucha. |
| Dinner | Fish, Vegetables, limited potatoes |
| Stretching | Day off |

# Day 2 - Variation Day

Some days it is not possible to fit in even a fifteen-minute workout but substituting for another activity while maintaining some focus on diet is also beneficial.

| | |
|---|---|
| Breakfast | Egg, Kefir & Berries. Coffee |
| Key mobility exercises | 9 of each (no timer) |
| Upper body and core | Rest day |
| Lower body | Rest day (more walking instead) |
| Lunch | Salad (spinach, lettuce, feta, chickpea, sunflower seeds, feta, steak) |
| Dinner | Anything |
| Stretching | All |

# Day 3 - Circuits Day

On days when you want to really push your overall fitness try to hit a variety of body weight exercises.

| | |
|---|---|
| Breakfast | Egg on toast. Coffee |
| Key mobility exercises | All |
| Upper body and core | Pull ups<br>Chin ups<br>Push ups<br>Archer push ups<br>V ups<br>Crunches<br>Flutter kicks |
| Lower body | Squats<br>Bosu Ball Squats<br>Lunge Squats with Kettlebell<br>Bosu Ball step up<br>Squats<br>Bosu Ball Squats |
| Lunch | Leftovers (food ordering vegetables, meat, starch). Apple cider vinegar drink. |
| Dinner | Anything |
| Stretching | Rest |

# Day 4 - Core Day

One day a week you should focus on exercises that primarily challenge your upper body and core strength.

| | |
|---|---|
| Breakfast | Kefir and Berries. Coffee. |
| Key mobility exercises | All |
| Upper body and core | Bosu ball push up<br>V up<br>Crunch<br>Flutter kicks<br>Bosu cross crunches<br>Pike Push Ups<br>Bosu Balance Crunch |
| Lower body | Assisted Front Kick<br>Assisted Back Kick<br>Assisted Side Kick<br>Single Leg Box Squat |
| Lunch | Leftovers (food ordering vegetables, meat, starch). Apple cider vinegar drink. |
| Dinner | Food ordering vegetables, meat, starch |
| Stretching | All |

# Day 5 - Legs Day

One day a week you should focus on developing leg strength and stability.

| | |
|---|---|
| Breakfast | Egg on toast. Coffee |
| Key mobility exercises | All |
| Upper body and core | V-up<br>Crunch<br>Push up<br>Band pull apart<br>Band arm curl<br>V-up<br>Flutter kicks |
| Lower body | Squats<br>Bosu Squats<br>Bosu Squats with kettlebell<br>Lunge squats with kettlebell<br>Bosu Squats<br>Squats |
| Lunch | Leftovers (food ordering vegetables, meat, starch). Apple cider vinegar drink. |
| Dinner | Anything |
| Stretching | All |

# Day 6 - Rest Day

It is OK to take a day off once a week. Rest is not just physical, but also mental, just remember not to completely overindulge.

| | |
|---|---|
| Breakfast | Anything. Coffee |
| Key mobility exercises | Day Off |
| Upper body and core | Day Off |
| Lower body | Day Off |
| Lunch | Anything |
| Dinner | Food ordering vegetables, meat, starch |
| Stretching | Day Off |

# Day 7 - Stretch Day

At least one day a week should be devoted to relaxing the muscles and working out the kinks in your body.

| | |
|---|---|
| Breakfast | Anything. Coffee |
| Key mobility exercises | Day Off |
| Upper body and core | Day Off |
| Lower body | Day Off |
| Lunch | Food ordering vegetables, meat, starch |
| Dinner | Food ordering vegetables, meat, starch |
| Stretching | All |

# Final Thoughts

This is my first book, and, as a busy person, it was not easy to write. I completed my primary objectives by:

- Framing the increasingly subtle environmental threats to living a healthy lifestyle
- Reviewing my own challenges of trying to exercise over a period of decades.
- Sharing my anecdotal exploration of maximizing my limited time and resources.
- Highlighting the key principles so that others can apply them.
- Providing a structured set of exercises and routines to enable a starting point.

I am also in the process of starting a YouTube and Facebook page for The Compact Workout and will add material there if the interest is significant enough. I may even write more in the future. At this point though it is up to you, dear reader. Are you a busy person, with often overwhelming responsibilities? Are you looking to get some control over your health and your sense of wellbeing? Are you ready to set realistic expectations and follow through with some simple but highly effective changes?

If you are this person, make a promise to yourself right now. That you will put down this book, find a timer (a configurable tabata timer on your phone works best), and do your first compact workout. And tomorrow you will do the same. And you will start eating a little better each day, and you will stretch a little each day, and you will keep going as far as you can. Be realistic in your goals, find opportunities each day, and adapt your exercise schedule around your obstacles. In this way you can achieve results you never considered and empower yourself in ways you never knew possible.

www.ingramcontent.com/pod-product-compliance
Lightning Source LLC
Chambersburg PA
CBHW050821250726

48653CB00006B/2348